Anxiety & Depression

Effective Strategies for Coping

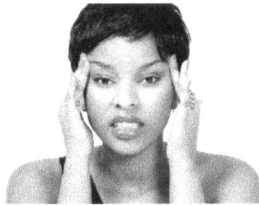

Sue Kennedy

Income Disclaimer

This document contains strategies, methods and other advice that, regardless of my own results and experience, may not produce the same results (or any results) for you. I make absolutely no guarantee, expressed or implied, that by following the advice below you will make any headway or improve your current situation, as there are several factors and variables that come into play regarding any given method.

Primarily, results will depend on the nature of your lifestyle, the condition of your lifestyle, the experience of the individual, situations and elements that are beyond your control.

As with any endeavor, you assume all risk related to the results based on your own discretion and at your own potential input.

Liability Disclaimer

By reading this document, you assume all risks associated with using the advice given below, with a full understanding that you, solely, are responsible for anything that may occur as a result of putting this information into action in any way, and regardless of your interpretation of the advice.

You further agree that our company cannot be held responsible in any way for the success or failure of your outcomes as a result of the information presented below. It is your responsibility to conduct your own due diligence regarding the safe and successful operation of your lifestyle if you intend to apply any of our information in any way to your life.

Terms of Use

ANXIETY AND DEPRESSION

EFFECTIVE STRATGIES FOR COPING

Table of Contents

INTRODUCTION

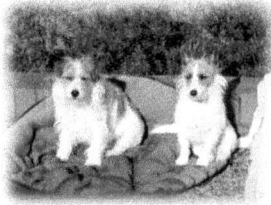

"A Champion is someone who gets up when he can't" - Jack Dempsey

Anxiety and depression is definitely not a nice thing to experience. A few years ago I had it all, husband, business, friends and my beautiful dog. What could go wrong? Everything was going to plan, our lives were finally on track with our goals and we were happy and successful.

I am not saying life was easy, because we worked hard, very hard; if you want to be successful this is a no brainer. As I said life was great and then one day it started - it slowly began to come crushing down all around me. I actually did not realise that I had anxiety and depression until it was nearly too late!

In the process of all this I made some very bad decisions and some good ones, but the good ones at the time did not help me overcome how I felt about my life. It all started with my marriage breakdown, and then not long after that I lost my beautiful dog that was the centre of my world, she really was my soul mate.

From this time on things went from bad to worse, I nearly lost my mum to Diabetes and then I had no job, no income and no-where to live, I was ready to give up.

How could things go so wrong, especially to me who is a very strong willed person that never lets anything get in my way of forging ahead – no matter how bad it is. I am telling you that our Almighty Creator put many difficult obstacles in front of me and there were quite a few times that I had had enough and I was ready to give up on me and my life.

And then one day out of the blue I met a lady that changed my life and gave me the hope that I needed to survive and move forward without looking back!

It was not easy, and it took me a while to get back on track with my life. I am glad I did not give up no matter how hard it got and I am truly grateful for each day of my life. So much beauty, and wonderful people surround me and I am thankful for taking that first step to the rest of my future!

I got through this and so can you! I have complete faith in you so please trust in yourself that you too will be fine and glow again!

I would really like to acknowledge a few people that really helped me get through this, and they probably don't even realise that they were a big part of me continuing on with my life; those people are:

My mum, my dear friend Sharen Shoard, and my business partner and friend John Flynn.

So I would like to take this opportunity to say thank you for your ongoing support, please know that I will be forever grateful.

Yours in Health & Gratitude,
Sue Kennedy

Chapter One

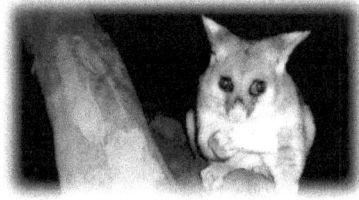

Understanding the signs of Anxiety & Depression

"Good humor is a tonic for mind and body. It is the best antidote for anxiety and depression. It is a business asset. It attracts and keeps friends. It lightens human burdens. It is the direct route to serenity and contentment." - Greenville Kleiser

Understanding the signs of anxiety and depression is a very real concern that should be taken seriously. Anxiety and depression are very real illnesses that can quickly take over your life. We tend to feel anxious on occasion and for some people, anxiety can sadly become a way of life and for many reasons that are unknown, even to the anxious person.

It is important to understand that anxiety has the ability to affect our entire body and mind. For people that struggle with anxiety it can change the way you feel, the way you behave, it can also affect your physical well-being.

Having anxiety is very much like feeling fear, and the worst part is that you may not even realise what you are fearful of or anxious about. What this causes is a nasty vicious cycle of feeling anxious and then you become afraid of being anxious.

Stress is a huge trigger for anxiety. Unfortunately we all suffer from stress at some point in our lives, and unfortunately some of us handle it quite differently to others.

The people that are not equipped to handle stress effectively find that they will struggle with anxiety.

Following are some of the symptoms anxiety may cause you:

- Headache
- Backache
- Numbness
- Muscle tension
- Upset stomach
- Rapid heart rate
- Increased perspiration
- Shaking
- Butterflies

It is very important to understand that depression is a very real condition. It is considered that depression is simply a state of mind and something that you should just "snap out of," it is very important that you realise that depression is an illness that affects not just your mind, but also your whole body.

When you are depressed you will experience changes in the way you sleep, eat, the way you feel about yourself, and even in the way you approach even the most mundane things in your life.

Please understand that depression is not just simply feeling "blue," it is a serious illness that can last weeks, months or even years.

If you are depressed, you will notice a variety of symptoms. These symptoms can and will vary from each individual and will also depend on the severity of the depression in each case.

Following are the experiences you may feel if you are depressed:

- Poor self esteem
- Thoughts of hurting yourself
- Difficulty focusing or making decisions
- Negative thought processes
- Feeling ill

- Getting better seems hopeless
- A lack of motivation or irritability
- Feelings of helplessness

Anxiety and depression are very serious illnesses that can quickly take over your life if you are not careful. The sad realisation is that you may not even notice how profoundly you are being affected by anxiety or depression.

The great news is that there are steps you can take to improve your physical and mental well-being if you suffer from anxiety or depression. Do not despair because there is a solution so that you can start improving your life starting today!

Chapter Affirmation:

I am climbing out of the pit of depression.

Life's tribulations may seem overwhelming, but I refuse to give up on myself. My life has a purpose and my happiness is worth fighting for. **I may fall, but I get up, dust off my shoes, and walk with steadfast determination.**

I refuse to succumb to the crippling effects of disappointment by accepting that things may not always work out the way I want them to. When things do not work out in my favor, I seek solutions.

In the face of difficult times, I pray and ask my Creator for guidance. The answers to my questions can be found through prayer. I protect my heart from bitterness when I accept the Creator's sovereign plan over my own.

In place of bitterness or self-pity, I embrace forgiveness. **Letting go of my hurt is the only way I can have a chance to live.** I forgive myself for my shortcomings and focus on my strengths. I forgive others for their role in contributing to any negative circumstances.

To keep loneliness far away, I surround myself with people who care about me. Having others rally around me is a source of comfort and strength. When I know I am not alone, I have the courage to stand up to depression.

The support of my friends and family is my lifeline. *Like a life raft, they support me. The unconditional love of those close to me helps me realise that there is more to life.*

Today, I choose life! I choose to embrace the healing love being offered to me so I may live a life filled with joy and purpose.

Self-Reflection Questions:

1. *Have I opened up to my loved ones about my feelings of depression?*
2. *Who can I lean on during difficult times?*
3. *What do I need to let go of and forgive myself for?*

20

Chapter Two

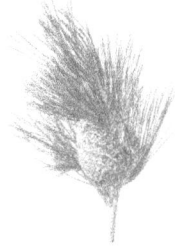

What are the different types of Anxiety?

"Nothing diminishes anxiety faster than action." - Walter Anderson

Many people do not realise that there are different types of anxiety, and by understanding the different types, it is much easier to learn how to deal with these.

It is also very important to realise that everyone experiences anxiety in a different way. There is a general anxiety that is easily managed but never goes away and then there is the anxiety that people experience in social situations. Understanding which type you suffer from is critical to find the right solutions for relief.

Anxiety is not a simple condition and it is not just nervousness that people encounter. Anxiety is both a physical and mental problem that affects millions of people worldwide.

Following are the seven categories of anxiety disorders:

- **General Anxiety Disorder (GAD)** – This type of disorder is the most common and has the essential characteristics of excessive worry and tension; a sense of fear even when there seems to be nothing or little to provoke that anxiety.

The most common symptoms associated with this type of anxiety are:

- o Irritation
- o Feeling of not being in control
- o Constant restlessness
- o Fatigue
- o General low energy levels
- o Tense muscles in your back, shoulders and neck
- o Unable to focus or concentrate on activities
- o Being obsessive over negative and anxious causing thoughts

- **Panic Disorder** – This type of anxiety is very different from GAD. Having a panic disorder is not about you being panicked; it is a disorder that you experience when you have severe feelings of doom and gloom that cause you both physical and mental symptoms, these become very intense and can cause hospitalisation in some cases. The symptoms of a panic disorder can include:

- o Heart palpitations
- o Sweating
- o Trembling and shaking
- o Heart racing
- o Chest pains
- o Sensation of shortness of breath
- o Feeling dizzy
- o Fear of dying
- o Numbness or tingling sensations
- o Digestive problems

Panic disorders generally end within ten minutes.

- **Obsessive Compulsive Disorder (OCD)** – It is understood that people with OCD continually have constant thoughts of fears that cause them to perform certain routines. They show behaviours and fears that seem unreasonable to those around them as well as to themselves. The difference between Obsessions and Compulsions are:

- o Obsessions are thought based, they are a preoccupied thought that is usually negative or fearful
- o Compulsions on the other hand are behaviour based, these are where the person "needs" to perform a certain activity or action.

- **Phobias** – This disorder is best described as the intense fear of a specific situation or object. Some phobias that people suffer from for example is the fear of birds also known as "Ornithophobia" or the fear of spiders is another one, known as "arachnophobia". A person with a phobia will go to extremes to avoid the situation or object in question, however it does cause extreme disruption to their lifestyles. If you notice that a phobia is starting to seriously affect your ability to live a good quality of life, then you need to seek professional treatment.

- **Social Anxiety Phobia** – This type of disorder is when someone is overwhelmed with worry and self-consciousness about every day social situations. The worry is usually focused on the fear of being judged by others or behaving in a way that may cause embarrassment or lead to ridicule.

It is normal to be shy in a social setting but when the shyness becomes intense and the idea of mixing in public, with strangers, or even your friends can be a sign of anxiety and fear associated with social phobia. People with social anxiety phobia often suffer from two or more of the following:

- o Intense issues when meeting new people
- o Obsessed about being watched or judged
- o A severe fear of public speaking
- o A feeling of hopelessness or fear with strangers or new situations
- o Becoming anxious at the thought of a social event, even when they are not in one
- o Difficulty coping in a social situation that makes you overwhelmingly anxious

- **Post Traumatic Stress Disorder (PTSD)** – This is an anxiety disorder that is developed after a traumatic or terrifying situation like a physical or sexual assault, the death of a loved one or a car accident. A person that suffers PTSD will in most cases need the help of a professional as this kind of disorder can affect you for years or possibly the rest of your life.

A person with PTSD will have regular instances of frightening and unwelcome thoughts, they will have a flashback of the event that occurred and when this happens the person feels like they are reliving the experience of the event.

- **Agoraphobia** – When you suffer from this disorder it is known as the fear of going out in public, it can be also the fear of open spaces or unfamiliar places. People that suffer from this disorder will do everything to avoid leaving their home.

It is understood that people who suffer agoraphobia also have panic disorder as agoraphobia is caused by panic attacks. Not everyone that suffers from agoraphobia spend all their time indoors, however, there are different levels, some of the more common symptoms are:

- Feeling tension and stress in normal regular activities like stepping outdoors, going to the shop or talking with strangers
- A complete obsessive fear of being in a social environment with people you know or do not know
- Feeling severe stress or anxiety when you are in an environment outside of your home where you have no control
- Allowing your fears to keep you prisoner and preventing you from living your life normally because of that fear

It does not matter which disorder you suffer from, as there is help out there for you. Once you recognise which disorder you suffer from it is important to choose a treatment that will help you deal with your disorder effectively.

Understanding your anxiety disorder and choosing an effective treatment will allow you to live your life with more control and happiness. Many people have been able to cure their anxiety disorder completely, while others find ways to make life easily manageable so that they can live a normal life once more.

Chapter Affirmation:

I have the power to change what I believe.

I recognise the impact my beliefs have on how I feel and behave. Believing something about a situation determines how events progress. What I think and feel about another person affects how I relate to that person. *My beliefs in myself determine how I perform.*

However, I can choose what I believe. **If I want to see a situation differently, I have the power to do so.**

My beliefs are particularly important when I am relating to others. If I believe a person has certain qualities, then I assume I know how they think and act. But when I change my mind about someone, I see the person differently, often for the better. I am free to determine what I believe about someone.

My beliefs about myself determine my level of confidence. Whether I am beginning a new project, attending a social event, or experiencing changes in a personal relationship, **how my life progresses is largely determined by what I believe.** And I am blessed with the power to change how I see things.

Knowing I can change what I believe brings success into my life. Inside myself, I make a decision about what I think is true. But if I observe factors that do not coincide with my beliefs, I change how I view other people and situations based on this new information.

Today, I plan to embrace my power to change my beliefs. I can alter those beliefs that ultimately result in less than ideal situations, relationships, or behavior.

Self-Reflection Questions:

1. Do I have the power to change my beliefs?
2. What is a particular assumption that hinders me?
3. How can I create more success by accepting my power to change my beliefs?

Chapter Three

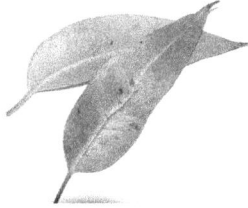

What Are The

Different Types Of

Depression?

"Happiness does not depend upon who you are or what you have. It depends solely upon what you think" –
Dale Carnegie

Depression is unfortunately more common these days than ever before. Depression is a psychological disorder that makes a person feel hopeless, sad, pessimistic, guilty, and worthless.

A person suffering from depression usually has difficulty concentrating or making any decisions, they have difficulty sleeping, have a lack of energy, a loss of appetite, and sometimes even show physical symptoms like slow movement or speech.

The most important point to remember is that depression must be taken seriously because sadly there is a very high rate of suicide associated with it.

Most people believe that there is only one type of depression, however, there a many types of depression, as you will see below.

Atypical Depression

This depression is a variation of depression that is a little different from Major depression. The person suffering from this is able to feel and experience happiness and moments of great pride and joy. The symptoms of atypical depression most commonly include:

- Weight gain
- Fatigue
- Overeating
- Oversleeping

A person that suffers atypical depression has the strong belief that the outside world controls their moods. This type of depression can last for many months or some people can live with it forever.

Major Depression

This type of depression is the most common form of all depressions. It is also common to know people that suffer from this type of depression. The typical symptoms of this type of depression are where a person goes around with the weight of the world on their shoulders. This person will not have any interest in getting involved in any regular activities and is completely convinced that they will remain in this state. These people will also lose their appetite, experience weight loss and lose interest in any sexual activities.

Dysthymia

People that suffer from dysthymia are usually not even aware that they suffer from this and continue to live their lives each day with a feeling of being sad and melancholic. These people don't enjoy their lives because they are always feeling dissatisfied, unimportant, or frightened. This type of depression requires the attention of a medical professional that can administer the right type of medication.

Post-Natal Depression

This type of depression is also known as the "baby blues", it affects on average about half of all new mothers. The symptoms of this type of depression can include:

- Mild depression
- Being tense or unwell
- Anxious
- Trouble sleeping

This type of depression can last from a few hours or a few days and then disappear. Mothers that suffer from post-natal depression find it increasingly difficult to cope with the demands of daily life.

Mothers can experience fear, anxiety, sadness, despondency, and extreme tiredness. Some may even suffer from a panic attack or become quite tense and irritable, a change in appetite and sleep patterns may also occur.

There is also a severe but rare case of post-natal depression known as puerperal psychosis. This is where a woman is unable to cope with her daily life and can become disturbed in the way she thinks and behaves.

It is very important for a mother and child that post-natal depression is treated by a professional.

Psychotic Depression

This is not a nice type of depression to suffer from, people start to hear and see imaginary things, and they hear sounds, voices and see things that do not exist.

This is called a hallucination that is commonly suffered by people with schizophrenia. Unfortunately, these hallucinations are not positive ones, as a manic-depressive would see them; they instead see images that are frightening that have negative sounds and images attached to them.

Manic Depression

This form of depression is known as the emotional disorder that can change your mood and shift it from depression to mania and this can often be quite rapid. This type of depression is also known as bipolar disorder. This must be taken seriously because sadly there is a very high rate of suicide associated with it.

It is very important that you seek professional help so that you can treat the correct type of depression.

Chapter Affirmation:

My life is an adventure.

Life is an amazing gift. From the miracle of conception to the mystery of the ever after, life is truly divine.

I am in charge of my life and I can choose what kind of life I lead. **It is up to me and only me to make my life whatever I want it to be.**

My life is an adventure. I choose to see my life as an exciting journey filled with highs and lows. The ups and downs of life are more fascinating than a Broadway play. The excitement of real life is incomparable.

Positive events in my life are sweet times during which I make memories that I can treasure for years to come. The good times serve as motivation during the not so good times to remind me that, once I get over the mountain, the ride will be smooth again.

During the low times in my life, I put on the armor of a positive outlook and charge forward. *Humor is the sword I use to cut through the tough times. I laugh at myself and at negative situations because laughing is better than crying.*

When I have a particularly crazy day, I take a deep breath and smile to myself thinking about how much fun the day was. In the end, easy days are boring; those crazy days are the ones that keep my life interesting.

Today, I choose to have a good attitude about life. ***I take the bad with the same joy as I take the good, because it is all part of the journey of life that I love so much.***

Self-Reflection Questions:

1. *How is my life an adventure?*
2. *How can I change my attitude about life?*
3. *How can I bring more fun into my life and my perspective?*

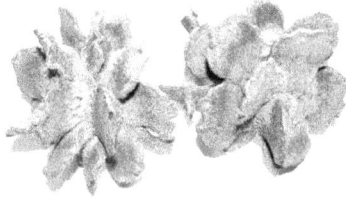

Chapter Four

Let's Get Down To The Real Issues

"Be miserable. Or motivate yourself. Whatever has to be done, it's always your choice" - Wayne Dyer

It's now time to take a good look at why you are suffering from anxiety and depression. If you are feeling sad or anxious, it could be because of what happened in your past. Taking a look at your past can provide you with many clues as to the origins of your current day problems.

It is important to take a look at your childhood and look at what your parents were like, what was your relationship like with them and any other early experiences you had that could contribute to your anxiety and depression. Reflecting on your past may bring about some very powerful emotions, so please stop this process if you start to feel overwhelmed and consult with a mental health professional for continued support and guidance.

Early experiences are not always the reason for your suffering, it can also be a culmination of events that build up and all come crashing down one after the other, this is fairly common with a lot of people. It is not easy dealing with one thing after another going wrong, hence why people fall into depression and become quite anxious.

Following are some questions that will help you establish why you are feeling the way you are today in your current life. Answer them as honestly as you can so that you can start to see a pattern form and work out why this is happening to you.

- What were your parents like?
- What kind of discipline did they implement?
- What was the relationship like with your parents?
- Were your parents supportive and a good guidance or were they critical of everything you did?
- Did your parents spend quality time with you?
- Do you have any negative or positive memories of your parents?
- Were there any significant reasons why your parents could not care for you properly, for example, a divorce, death, work, travel or illness?
- If you have siblings, were there any problems that you can recall?
- Were you happy at school?
- Was there anything significant that stood out at school that caused emo-

tional scarring, for example, bully-
ing?
- What were your friendships like while growing up?
- Have you had any major setbacks or traumas in your life?

Once you have answered these questions, take a look and see if you can pinpoint why you are suffering from anxiety and depression. The important point to re-member is that it is not your fault, there is always a reason why you are going through this, by finding this reason you can start to resolve the situation and start enjoying your life once more.

Chapter Affirmation:

I live my life for today.

I live my life for today without worries of what may happen tomorrow. The little time I have to spend with my family and friends is valuable, so I squeeze out every last drop of enjoyment as I go.

*Playing with my children, spending romantic evenings with my spouse, and laughing with family is what it is all about. **I am fortunate to have such a rewarding life** and it is only right that I pay my reality the attention it deserves.*

*Though I plan for a better tomorrow, I cannot allow my dreams and aspirations to interfere with my present. I work hard to obtain what I desire. **It would be a shame to miss savoring the fruits of my labor.***

I refuse to concern myself with past events or things yet to come. Holding grudges is a waste of energy and daydreaming takes my focus away from the wonderful life I already have. I deserve to enjoy the hours as they pass without worries or distractions.

I live everyday as if it were my last. *My insecurities, fears, hopes, and dreams are irrelevant to this moment. I live my* life in the now and I am free from the regrets of yesterday.

Today, I enjoy each moment for what it is. I hug, kiss, and spend time with my loved ones regardless of what they may have done yesterday or may do tomorrow. Today is my day to live!

Self-Reflection Questions:

1. Do my aspirations prevent me from enjoying my current reality?
2. Is my regret from years past still haunting me?
3. How can I create more time to do things that I enjoy?

Chapter Five

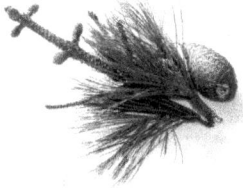

Recognising The Hurdles In The Way Of Change

"Desire is the starting point of all achievement, not a hope, not a wish, but a keen pulsating desire which transcends everything" - Napoleon Hill

By recognising the hurdles in the way of change is vitally important for you to conquer. I am certain that you do not wish to feel anxious or depressed all the time, you would like to take action about your situation but perhaps you feel incapable or overwhelmed just by the thought of it, am I right?

Please understand that there is something you can do to overcome this feeling, however please remember that at times there will be situations that are beyond your control. The situations that you can control can be overcome by understanding and overcoming those hurdles that get thrown in your way, your mind will try to prevent you from moving forward, so all you need to do is take action regardless.

It is important to realise that everyone views change in different ways. Some people find change scary, and some truly believe that they do not deserve to be happy at all which sadly means that these people will make no attempt at all to change.

Having these assumptions can be a hurdle that will get in the way of change and will keep you in a state of anxiety and depression. Some people are unaware that they have these assumptions and therefore it will interfere with their progress of moving forward with change.

If you have tried to make changes in the past and have failed, it will more than likely be because one of these assumptions are responsible. You cannot just sweep these under the door, you need to deal with these assumptions and realise what they are, plus you need to firmly believe and declare that you no longer believe in them. The way you deal with this situation is to restructure the way you think.

Chapter Affirmation:

I live a life free from worry and fear.

*I am brave and courageous, and I can do anything I put my mind to. **Fear and worry pass me by because I am strong.** I refuse to allow worries and* *fears to bother me or make a home in my thoughts.*

I know I have control over my own destiny, and I choose to move into that destiny boldly and without hesitation. Running away solves nothing! I work toward my goals with courage and perseverance, creating a destiny of success.

Worries and fears are absent from my life. I let the past stay in the past, without regrets or worries to cloud my present. I focus on the wonders of each new day and I shrug off fear about the future, since I trust that good things will come. I am happy, content, and brave.

I take on tasks with strength and courage. I can accomplish my dreams because I bravely take chances and try new things that can push me forward toward my goals.

Regardless of what comes my way, I can handle it. Rather than fearing things I don't understand, I learn the facts I need to ease my concerns. No weapon formed against me can prosper, as **I am capable of overcoming any challenge.** I banish fear, seek solutions, and boldly take action to get back on track.

Shedding the shackles of worry and fear gives me the freedom to live with all the gusto I've got so I can enjoy my life to the fullest!

Today, I plan to be brave, courageous, and bold in everything I do.

Self-Reflection Questions:

1. How can I move forward more boldly in my life?
2. What does being brave and courageous do for me?
3. What can I accomplish if I don't let fear and worry stop me?

54

Chapter Six

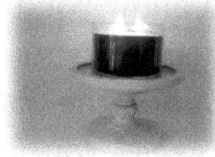

Understanding & Dealing With Your Moods

"Don't wish it were easier, wish you were better" - Jim Rohn - Mark Twain

It is important that you understand how your moods react to your body's response to certain situations. Knowing this information will help you become aware of the physical components of anxiety and depression.

Making a list of your feelings and then identifying them to different circumstances will allow you to become aware of the connection between the feelings, situations and the body sensations which will give you a better understanding of your moods.

Keep a record of your body responses and note down any significant reactions to each of these, as well as what you were doing at the time. This information will help you connect between situations and the responses to each.

Following are some examples of a body response:
- Headaches
- Breathing
- Fatigue
- Muscle tightness
- Posture
- Stomach symptoms
- Light-headed
- Restless legs
- Dizziness

- Disorientation
- Tingling
- Constriction in throat or chest

Your body will give you signals and once you understand these you can connect them to your mental and physical state.

Following is a list of feeling words for you to help identify your feelings. Each day write down your feelings from this list. By using this list you will be able to give your mental and physical state a feeling name, which will allow you to connect your feelings with your body sensations and know which situation triggered it.

Fear	Anger
Nervous	Annoyed
Afraid	Irritable
Tense	Bitter
Worried	Resentful
Terrified	Furious
Apprehensive	Mad
Timid	Outraged
Panic	Livid

Shame	Sadness
Embarrassed	Heartache
Disgraced	Distressed
Guilty	Anguish
Humiliation	Grief
Degraded	Sorrow
Chagrin	Hopeless
Remorse	Miserable
Mortification	Dispirited

Chapter Affirmation:

My life gets better every day.

*My life is on an upward swing. Each new day is more rewarding than the day before as my life flourishes. **I am rich in blessings and relationships because I have aligned myself on the path of abundance.***

Life is a progression of actions and results of those actions. My actions and choices are yielding for me a plethora of benefits. My cup overflows with joy in the harvest of the seeds I plant.

I remain focused and motivated by keeping my goals in sight. Even in times of sorrow, I continue pressing on so that I may enjoy the fruit of my labor in the future.

To encourage myself, I recall situations where I was successful. ***Knowing that I have previously conquered my fears reassures me that my future is filled with triumph.***

As I look at my past and reflect on its lessons, I equip myself with strength and wisdom. The more I live, the more I learn. I grow as an individual with each bit of knowledge I apply to my current situation.

Today, I choose to fill my heart with the expectation of great things to come. Even as I cherish the abundance of the present, I believe that my best day is ahead of me.

Self-Reflection Questions:

1. *How is my life today better than it was yesterday?*
2. *What am I looking forward to in the future?*
3. *Why is it necessary for me to choose hope?*

Chapter Seven

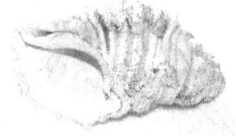

Looking At

Everything

Differently

"People become really quite remark-
able when they start thinking that
they can do things. When they believe
in themselves they have the first
secret of success" - Norman Vincent
Peale

In this chapter I would like to discuss
Cognitive Behavioural Therapy (CBT) and

how this treatment is a focused approach for different types of behavioural, emotional and psychiatric conditions. The form of CBT that is introduced to the person will vary according to the situation that requires attention.

It is a program that is tailored for each individual to help identify any bad behaviours or thoughts so that help can be given to change and teach you how to re-introduce good behaviours and thoughts.

CBT has been researched very extensively for more than thirty years and has proven to be very effective in the treatment of many psychological emotions and psychiatric problems.

The principle of Cognitive Behavioural Therapy is best described as changing how you behave that will lead to changes in what you think and feel.

There are occasions when you will have distortions in your thinking. When this happens, you are not able to accurately reflect, predict or describe what is happening. This kind of distorted thinking can become a terrible problem, especially if it ends up in anxiety or depression.

The three main types of distortion are as follows:

- Self-blaming reality distortions
- Incoming information reality distortions
- Self-judging reality distortions

To recognise self-blaming reality distortions you will blame yourself for everything and place all the blame for wrongdoing on yourself.

The best way to describe incoming information reality distortions is the different ways that your mind will distort the information that is coming in.

Self-judging is a form of self-sabotage which effects the way you view your be-

63

haviour and yourself. Unfortunately, anxious and depressed states of mind become very judgemental, harshly critical and self-derogatory.

Distorted perceptions can actually trigger a cycle of anxious feelings that can lead to an anxiety disorder. Some of these perceptions are:

- Seeing a mildly threatening situation as extremely dangerous
- Looking at yourself as being incapable of self-protection
- Inability to see real and immediate dangers
- Believing that an unidentified danger will occur
- See every situation or person as a threat
- Having the belief that danger is unavoidable and inevitable

Chapter Affirmation:

I stay positive when circumstances seem grim.

Reality is more than just my perception. The truth is what I choose to believe about what I perceive. The eyes of my soul see clearly through the lens of faith, regardless of what my physical eyes see.

When the world around me gets grim, I stay calm because the eyes of faith allow me to see beyond apparent circumstances. Although I may initially perceive negativity, **I find something positive in every situation.**

A dead end to most people is the beginning of a new opportunity for me to be creative. When I face an obstacle, I immediately pray for peace of mind. My ability to have a positive attitude in times of crisis begins with inner peace.

Prayer is more than just a last resort when I have run out of options; it is the first place I turn.

Through the darkest of times, I find comfort in knowing that there is enough grace for me to walk through whatever situation I experience.

I can be positive in the midst of grim circumstances because **I focus on the lesson to be learned, rather than the price to be paid.** I am thankful for the difficult moments in life because those are the ones that help me grow.

Today, I choose to be a ray of hope in the darkness by finding any trace of positivity and magnifying it. I turn to prayer as my lifeline even when I would rather succumb to my fears.

Self-Reflection Questions:

1. What lesson can I learn from the situations I find myself in today?
2. What is the role of prayer in adjusting my attitude?
3. How is perception a choice? What do I choose to see when I look at my life?

Chapter Eight

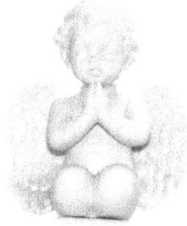

The Ability To

Challenge & Change

Your Thoughts

"Issue a blanket pardon. Forgive everyone who has ever hurt you in any way. Forgiveness is a perfectly selfish act. It sets you free from the past" – Brian Tracey

It can be a real challenge to find a way to turn negative thoughts into positive ones and sometimes it takes more than just medication. Depression is a huge challenge because of how it can change the way you think.

For people that do not suffer from depression, they too can have many negative and positive thoughts throughout the day; however, if you suffer from depression then you will filter the world through negative thoughts to the extent that it will distort reality and the overall outlook on your life. People with depression will view the world quite differently.

The biggest challenge people with depression have is that they get caught in a dangerous spiral that leads to negative thinking and that negative thinking makes them even more depressed.

Unfortunately negative thinking for many can become a habit that they use as a defence technique for coping with the symptoms of depression.

The ability to change your thoughts is done by re-training your brain with positive thoughts. This of course will not happen overnight, it will take a lot of practice as well as the help of a professional.

Here are some tips to help you with your mindset and help you with changing your thoughts into positive ones:

- Cognitive therapy – this is a very effective treatment for depression; a therapist can help you understand, recognise and find ways to undo your negative thinking.
- Relaxing – it is important to take time out to relax each day for a few minutes, this can be done by some deep breathing, meditation or yoga. This can be extremely helpful when your thoughts or emotions start to get out of control.
- Write – get yourself a notebook where you can write down all your negative thoughts, this can be very beneficial in helping you find a more

rational and positive way to think about things. Listing all these negative thoughts can help you see a pattern that will emerge so that you can understand what triggered those negative thoughts so that you can find ways to change them.

- Overall health – It is very important that you maintain a healthy lifestyle, limit your alcohol intake, exercise on a regular basis and eat well, all these will lead to a positive outcome as well as positive thoughts.

Chapter Affirmation:

Worries are easy for me to handle.

There will always be worries in life. How I handle those worries is up to me, and I choose to handle them well.

*Worries are easy for me to deal with because I know bothersome situations are only temporary. **Worries always pass so I allow them to float away.***

*I am strong, brave, and able to dispel worries with a single thought. Instead of worrying over things, I make plans to overcome any challenges I see. I move forward confidently, without fear or concern. **I know I can handle my life.***

Anything that comes my way is okay, because I know I can deal with life. I accept the twists and turns that life gives me. I find ways to make lemons into lemonade, and use any worries to spur me forward rather than hinder me.

*I make bold choices and take reasonable risks. I get ahead in life and accomplish my dreams and goals. **I refuse to be held back by fear.** Moving forward bravely is the only way to go and it is the way I choose to live my life.*

*I am comfortable with the way my life is working out. I know all things are for my ultimate good, even if they are scary at the time. **I am brave and strong** and I can conquer my worries each day.*

Today, I release all my fears and worries and accept only peace and joy.

Self-Reflection Questions:

1. *How can I have fewer worries in my life?*
2. *What can I do to stay positive in any situation?*
3. *How can I encourage others to let go of their fears and worries?*

Chapter Nine

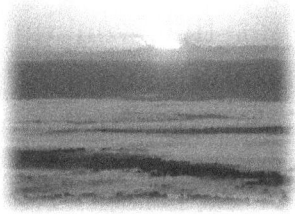

Being Able To See Through The Fog

"The secret of health for both mind and body is not to mourn for the past, not to worry about the future, not to anticipate troubles, but to live in the present moment wisely and earnestly" - Buddha

There are different treatments for anxiety and depression and depending on what your condition is will determine how you should get it treated. The best way is for you to seek the advice of a professional and learn all the different treatments that are available.

It is important that you understand all these options and then you can discuss with your therapist which treatment will fit your specific situation.

There are conventional treatments for depression and anxiety as well as lifestyle changes that are highly recommended.

It is of interest to note that anxiety will precede depression, usually by several years and on average it happens in your late childhood/early adolescence years. It is also important to realise that a young person is not likely to outgrow anxiety if it does not get treated with cognitive therapy.

If you apply an aggressive treatment for your anxiety issues when they occur, it is highly likely that you can prevent the development of depression.

There is help available for everyone, so please understand that you are not alone and that you can get through this, and please realise that you cannot do this alone, you will need someone to help you every step of the way. I want you to make sure that if you need help that you ask for it.

People get caught up in their own worlds and may not realise that you need help, so please alert them; they are there to help.

So that you can see through the fog, you must first stop all those negative thoughts and replace them with healthy positive and truthful thoughts. If you work hard each day to implement these positive thoughts you will see the light at the end of the tunnel.

Cognitive therapy is actually focused at ten common distortions or faulty thought patterns that can send you into a depression, these are as follows:

- Overgeneralising
- Jumping to conclusions
- Emotional reasoning
- Disqualifying the positive
- All or nothing thinking
- Mental filter
- Labelling and mislabelling
- Personalisation
- Magnification and minimisation, and
- Should statements

Chapter Affirmation:

I can overcome depression.

I am defined by the actions I take in response to depression and not by the depression itself. I am defined by my personality, my actions, and my beliefs. I define myself!

I am stronger than these feelings of depression. I know that deep within myself, I have the ability to stop these feelings. In fact, I am so in control of my emotions that I can turn a negative into a positive using only the power of my mind.

I find that thinking factually rather than emotionally is the most effective method of ridding my heart of these feelings of depression. Generally, **I can shift my mood from depressed to contentment within just a matter of minutes.**

For example, when I begin to feel lonely, I remind myself that loving people surround me. And, when I feel an overwhelming impending sense of doom, I remind myself that both my loved ones and I are safe. I feel grateful for my blessings and find that **this thankful feeling is my best weapon against depression!**

Overall, I am a happy person. I live an exciting lifestyle, surrounded by loving people, and I am a successful professional.

*I understand that every now and then, everyone encounters a small bout of sadness. And generally, the **negative emotions are brought about by a sense of insecurity or an underlying worry.***

Today, I overcome my depression by accepting my emotions and then focusing my thoughts on something positive. I am a powerful, independent and stable individual. A small bout of sorrow is simply a small inhibition that I can overcome if I apply myself.

Self-Reflection Questions:

1. *Is there a specific person, place or thing that serves as a trigger?*
2. *Have I contacted my doctor about treatment?*
3. *Do I express my feelings, or keep them to myself?*

Chapter Ten

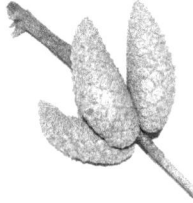

The Importance Of Mindfulness

"Learn the art of patience. Apply discipline to your thoughts when they become anxious over the outcome of a goal. Impatience breeds anxiety, fear, discouragement and failure. Patience creates confidence, decisiveness and a rational outlook, which eventually leads to success." - Brian Adams

What is mindfulness? Sit for a few minutes quietly with your eyes closed and just pay attention to your breathing. Now just feel the air as it passes through your nostrils and fills your lungs and then concentrate on the sensation as you exhale and you feel your lungs deflating.

If a thought appears in your mind, take note of them as if you were an observer and allow them to float on by, then focus back on your breathing.

This breathing exercise is an introduction to mindfulness. Mindfulness is best described as the state of awareness of the present, in the absence of any judgement, analysis or reasoning.

Another way to explain this is by calling it awareness; without thinking about your thinking or entering into a conversation with your thoughts. Once you get the hang of acceptance; this involves tolerance, patience and the willingness to feel and experience what it is to have no resistance. This is how you achieve mindfulness.

Mindfulness is also a technique that can be used to help you pay attention and be able to cope with everyday life, it will help you through the tough times which will benefit your physical and mental health.

An easy way to remember what mindfulness means is to:
- Focus on the present
- Pay attention, and
- Not worrying about the past or the future

Mindfulness is being recognised as another effective way to help people with their feelings, to be able to effectively handle painful thoughts, reduce stress, and increase self-awareness and emotional intelligence.

There are many benefits to implementing mindfulness:

- Decrease depression
- Decrease anxiety
- Be less moody or angry

- Be much happier
- Better sleeping habits
- Better breathing
- Better mechanisms to cope with pain
- Be more emotionally stable
- Better memory
- Improvement on your circulation
- Lowering of heart rate
- Better immune system
- Experience more calm and peace
- Experience unpleasant thoughts and feelings much easier
- Have more balance with your emotions
- Understand that your thoughts and feelings come and go, and
- Develop self-compassion and self-acceptance

Chapter Affirmation:

My cheerful attitude infuses joy wherever I go.

Wherever I go, I bring a smile with me because joy is part of who I am. **I am happy because I choose to see life through appreciative eyes.** *I focus on my blessings so I can be happy with my life.*

There is nothing more beautiful than a smiling face. Regardless of the circumstances I encounter, the joy that is within me is reflected through my actions. **Happiness is an attitude,** *and it is up to me.*

If I want to be surrounded by positive people, I must eliminate negativity from my own life. People around me are inevitably injected with my joy. My cheerful attitude is contagious.

When I speak, my words are filled with cheer and encouragement. I make people feel comfortable when they are close to me by being friendly, patient, and easy going. My personality draws other positive people.

To be joyful, I focus on solutions instead of problems. *I maintain an optimistic mood about the future. Having a cheerful attitude is a powerful tool in creating success. I confidently expect to succeed and my expectations become my reality.*

*I stimulate my creativity and generate opportunities for personal growth when I choose a positive perspective. **A positive outlook on life can change the entire view.** As a result of my attitude, I enjoy vibrant health.*

Today, I choose to bring joy with me wherever I go. I share my happiness with others through positive speech and kind gestures.

Self-Reflection Questions:

1. *What are the benefits of a joyful attitude?*
2. *How can I be more positive?*
3. *How do I make those around me feel?*

Chapter Eleven

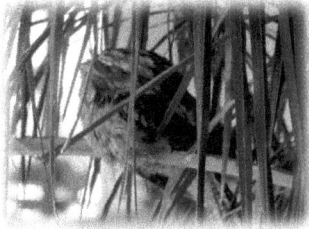

Stand Up To Your Fears

"Every tomorrow has two handles. We can take hold of it with the handle of anxiety or the handle of faith"
- Henry Ward Beecher"

How does fear relate to anxiety and depression? Surprisingly, it is related quite closely; when you are feeling anxious it is usually because you are reacting to something that you fear. The unfortunate part is that if this situation keeps occurring then it leads to depression.

Firstly, you need to identify what your fear is before you can stand up to it. Make a list of what fears you have, then write next to that fear what sets off that fear; by keeping a journal of these, you can easily identify what these fears are and then decide on how you will deal with them.

Some fears can be ignored, for example, if heights are fearful to you, then you simply avoid places where there are heights. However, there are certain fears that you need to stand up to so that you can avoid the nasty consequences.

Following is an example of social anxiety, which is quite a common fear for many people.

Social anxiety is something that many people have experienced at some point in their lives. Being in a crowd surrounded by many people can be quite an intimidating situation, especially if you are a shy person to begin with.

The good news is that social anxiety can be overcome. Of course everyone is different, but you can change the way you respond to big crowds or unfamiliar people. By implementing the right strategies, you will be able to cope the next time you are confronted with this situation.

Following are some tips that can help you with your social anxiety:

1. **Practice makes perfect.** If you are someone that does not have many social engagements, then you are not giving yourself the opportunity to overcome your fear. The best solution is to find a small group that you can start to interact with, once you are comfortable with that, move onto bigger groups of people.

2. **Be yourself.** It is important to be you, not someone you think people want you to be. People want to get to know you, so make the people around you feel comfortable by being you and ask

them some questions. They will open up to you and then the conversation will begin and you will feel more comfortable as the conversation continues.

- **Remember that people are less concerned about your flaws than you are.** Understandably, social occasions can be quite overwhelming, especially if you are trying really hard to make it work. Remember, it is OK to make mistakes, when you do, simply laugh it off and those around you will feel at ease also. The people around you will feel just as intimidated because they do understand that people make mistakes.

3. **Talk it out.** It is really important that you discuss your struggles with this, either with a loved one or a good friend. Remember, if you need to then please ask for help, there is always someone that will be only too happy to help you. If your social anxiety is much more

complicated, then it is advisable that you contact a professional. Get help, don't let this fear take over your life – you deserve to enjoy the company of others without fear.

4. **Look on the bright side.** Remember to always look at every situation as good. If you are in a social surrounding and you are fearful – it is much easier to face your fears head-on. Take a look at your surroundings; chances are that you can find something about the situation that makes you smile. Once you get into the swing of things, your fears will shrink.

5. **Take steps to relax.** If you begin to panic, try to relax. Excuse yourself for a few moments to be alone. Take a few slow, deep breaths from your stomach. Continue breathing slowly and deeply as you return to the social situation. You'll feel confident and more in control when you breathe deeply.

6. **Join a group or club.** It is amazing how groups and clubs can be great places to practice social interaction with others who share the same interests that you do. There are many groups in all local areas, simply find one that interests you, and remember, if one group does not work, try another. By joining groups that you are passionate about will make conversations much easier.

Remember that your attitude and will to change makes all the difference. Get off the sidelines, pick a social situation you'd normally avoid, and use these strategies to overcome your fears. Turn social situations into opportunities to learn, grow, and experience all that life has to offer.

<u>**Chapter Affirmation:**</u>

There is great joy in the little things in life.

Little things make me laugh and bring me great joy. Joyous events of great magnitude make me happy, of course, but the small events add up in life and become the foundation of what brings me happiness and peace.

I partake in the little joys that happen around me each day. My baby's smile, my puppy's exuberance, and even the aroma of my morning coffee bring me happiness. If I look around, I can always find something to be joyful about in that moment.

Joy is a choice. *Because I know I control my own destiny, I choose to be joyful and happy.*

By taking joy from the little things, I am rarely disappointed. There is always something nearby that makes me happy. I like to live a simple life where small things matter each day. I share that philosophy and my joy with other people, so they can have joy in their lives.

By sharing my joy of little things with others, I am even happier. The joy I send out radiates back to me in everything I do. People appreciate my simple joy. **People find more joy in their own lives when I am around.**

I show people how to appreciate the little things in life, and it makes their lives better. By working to make my life more joyful, I am able to share more joy with others. **There is great power in great joy.**

Today, I take the time to reflect on the little things in life that make me smile.

Self-Reflection Questions:

1. *How can I find more joy in small things?*
2. *What can I do to show others how much joy is available to them?*
3. *Are there ways I can share more of my joy with others?*

Chapter Twelve

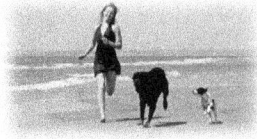

Exercise To Lift Your Spirits

"If you want to conquer the anxiety of life, live in the moment, live in the breath" - Amit Ray

Most people believe that the only way to fight depression is through therapy and medication, not so! Research has found that physical activity will increase the production and release of the naturally occurring feel good endorphins. (Endorphin means morphine produced naturally in the body).

It's true! Physical activity can have a profound impact on your ability to overcome what ails you because when your brain releases endorphins, you get a sense of well-being and pleasure. If you're feeling depressed, it might be time to incorporate exercise into your lifestyle.

There are many different types of exercise that you can implement. Please ensure that you check with your doctor before implementing any exercise regime to make sure it will not harm you. It is important to find exercises that will help you as well as suit your lifestyle.

Following are some effective strategies to fight depression with exercise:

1. **Experience the runner's high.** After a good workout, your body will experience what is known as a runner's high, this results from an endorphin surge in your body. The temporary

mood lift that this endorphin surge provides can be beneficial in reducing depression on a short-term basis.

- ***When you're feeling tense, overwhelmed, or down in general, seek a temporary pick me up in the form of a workout.*** This is when a short walk, hopping on a treadmill or riding your bike can be beneficial. Other ways you can boost your endorphins is to pick your mood up by doing some yoga, pilates or a strength-training workout.

- Exercise for at least 30 minutes per day can help you alleviate the symptoms of depression as well as providing you with a boost in your energy levels and concentration, this can help you reduce the negative feelings that are associated with depression.

2. **Improve your overall well-being.** Improving your health is very important and another way you can reduce your symptoms of depression is by implementing a strength training session in your exercise regime. An example of this is the lifting of dumbbells, it can help you build muscle, which helps to improve your metabolism and at the same time builds a stronger and healthier body.

   • While strength training may not directly impact your depression symptoms, its ability to improve your health can have long-term effects on your overall well-being.

3. **Exercise daily.** It is important to exercise each day for at least 30 minutes. According to the Journal of Preventive Medicine, several weeks after you establish this regular exercise routine, *you'll begin to feel relief of your depression symptoms on a much more consistent basis.*

4. **Replace medications with exercise.** The Journal of Preventive Medicine recently featured a study of patients with depression who worked out for at least 3 hours per week. This study found that the remission of these patients' symptoms was comparable to cognitive behavioral therapies and medication treatments.

- While exercise may not be able to completely replace your need for other treatment options, it is important to realise that it can benefit your mental well-being in many ways, making it an ***excellent way to balance the therapies that you rely on for relief.***

- Please make sure that if you are currently in treatment or taking medication, discuss any changes in therapy or medications with your doctor ***before*** you change them.

5. **Develop a routine.** It is easier than you think to develop a regular routine for exercise, and by doing so can have numerous benefits. Not only will you be controlling your depression with exercise itself, but also having a routine to look forward to can boost your spirits and ward off the overwhelming feelings of depression.

The Bottom Line

Depression can negatively impact your life in many ways. It will be very beneficial to you to experiment with different therapies and treatment options to make sure you get the help you need. Exercise is a great way to reduce the symptoms associated with depression: helping to clear your mind and improve your energy, while also giving you a general sense of well-being.

If you don't already have a regular exercise routine and you're suffering from depression, then *this is a treatment option that is well worth consider-*

ing. The results might surprise you! It may also work well in conjunction with current treatment options you are undertaking or it may replace those treatment options altogether. Please consult with your physician to learn more.

<u>Chapter Affirmation:</u>

My life is full of joy, health, and happiness.

My life is filled with everything good. Inside my heart there is an overabundance of positive emotions. When I think about my life, I am overwhelmed with gratitude for all my blessings. ***True joy is the result of a grateful heart.***

There are innumerable sources of joy in my life. My family and friends are the most precious gifts I have ever received. The unconditional love that I experience with them, especially in times of need, fill my heart with joy.

My joy is contagious and constant. **I choose to rejoice in every circumstance.** *I am filled with joy because I focus on the good things and give thanks for my life.*

The quality of my life matters; therefore I strive to live the best life I can. My goal is not merely to survive, but to live out the plan that has been set before me.

I practice healthy habits in order to enjoy good health. Good health improves my stamina and my ability to enjoy life. When I feel good physically, I feel good emotionally.

Everywhere I look, I see a new source of happiness. **I pay attention to the little details that make life great.**

Each day, I aim to share a deep laugh with someone. I allow myself to release my inhibitions, throw my head back, and laugh like a child. I surround myself with happy people in order to keep the feeling alive.

Today, I choose to look at life through appreciative eyes that focus on the small things that bring me joy, health, and happiness.

Self-Reflection Questions:

1. *What are my sources of joy?*
2. *How do I take care of my body?*
3. *What am I grateful for today?*

102

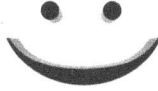

Chapter Thirteen

The Importance Of Having Fun

"Through laughter, a lot of the time you can defuse the tension that would usually be there" - Michael Hunter

Laughter has many benefits, especially for your health and well-being. Everyone enjoys a good laugh and there are different ways to enjoy this laughter, whether it is from your friends making a fool of themselves, watching a comedy show on TV or a live comedy show. When was the last time you had a good belly laugh? One that makes you cry and your bellyache!

If you are one of those people that find it hard to relax, then you'll be surprised that there are real benefits to having a good laugh. Yes, it does sound crazy, however it is true that your favourite TV show can do wonders for your health!

So how can laughter help you?

When you laugh, your body releases endorphins into the blood system. These endorphins act like natural painkillers and are also responsible for making you feel happy. The best part is endorphins are completely free of any side effects; it's all-natural! That's why you feel a "natural high" after the right dose of laughter.

Laughing not only leads to a feeling of well-being, but it can also help with the following:

- Lower blood pressure - This cycle starts with the blood pressure rising when you start to laugh but then it decreases to levels below normal. As you take deep breaths while laughing, more oxygen-rich blood is transported quickly throughout your body.

- Reduce stress and increase your attentiveness, heart rate and pulse - When your heart rate and pulse is elevated, you'll feel more energised. Of course, being more attentive can lead to better learning and growth.

- Make your heart grow stronger - For many years, heart specialists have established that mental stress is particularly harmful to the heart and is one of the leading causes behind the build up of fat and cholesterol in the coronary arteries. By laughing and reducing that stress on a regular basis, you're helping your body reduce that fat build-up while reducing your risk of a heart attack.

- Lower blood sugar - Laughter helps with reducing stress and stress often leads to an increase in blood sugar levels.

Laughter is a Form of Exercise!

You know when you throw back your head and laugh; you're actually working your muscles from the hips to your shoulders. And since laughing involves taking in and releasing of air, the expelling of carbon dioxide and the intake of oxygen, your internal organs and core muscles get a good workout every time you laugh heartily. It may sound silly, but it's true.

- Ever heard of "laughter yoga?" It's a form of a yoga class where you perform the regular stretches while doing silly things to induce laughter. Some of these activities include imitating animals to speaking in gibberish. If you think this sounds odd, you're right! It is. But we have to stop taking life so seriously and start having fun!

How You Can Improve Your Mental Health With Laughter?

Everyday you're faced with challenges and it's completely up to you how to confront them. There are two things you can do; you can choose a positive attitude or a negative one.

Remember that laughing when faced with a challenge can help lift your mood (as well as those around you) and one important point here is that maybe you'll be able to view the challenge in a positive light and not a negative one. This will help you reduce the stress and get things done quicker.

- When you laugh it is almost always followed by a sense of relaxation, and this is why it is a good form of stress relief.

- It is important to use laughter as a way to reconnect with your family, especially during troubling times.

107

Remember that when you laugh you generally talk more, as well as make direct eye contact; you even get into closer contact, which is a wonderful achievement.

A Laugh a Day Is Beneficial

As you can see, laughter has many physical benefits to your overall health and well-being, however it is very important that you exercise, have a healthy nutritious diet, and go for routine checkups. Nevertheless, there are simply many good reasons to laughing and it will help you enjoy the great fun life brings you and all that surrounds you as well!

Chapter Affirmation:

I radiate joy, love, and light.

I know I handle my life well because I am happy. I share that happiness with others, each and every day of my life. **Because I bring joy to others, joy,**

love, and light come back to me. *I take it all in and use these gifts to bless others whom I meet each day.*

I have love in my life. People are good to me, and I return that goodness to them through a kind word or gentle touch. Whatever people need, I help them feel better, and that brings me immeasurable joy and peace.

There is light in my life, and darkness fades away. The light is bright and beautiful, and it envelops everything I do. **Because the light is there for me, I use it to give light to others who may see only darkness in their lives.**

Darkness stays away from my life because it sees that it has no hold over me. I refuse to let problems bother me. I maintain my joy and peace through any trials that may appear. Challenges seem small to me because they lack power to affect me negatively.

My power goes only to love and light. It is used only to bring joy to others and myself. Negativity has no place in my life. I allow only good thoughts and kind people to be a part of my life.

Today, I let my joy, love, and light radiate out bright and strong, to touch the lives of others.

Self-Reflection Questions:

1. How can I bring more joy into my life today?
2. What can I do to share my joy with other people?
3. Who can I touch with my healing love and light today?

Chapter Fourteen

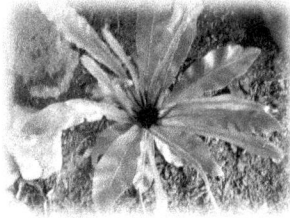

Dealing With

Problems Head On

"Self-pity gets you nowhere. One must have the adventurous daring to accept oneself as a bundle of possibilities and undertake the most interesting game in the world: making the most of one's best" – Harry Emerson Fosdick

Anxiety and depression can suck out all your energy; motivation and hope, especially when you are experiencing negative thoughts and emotions. You tend to find it very hard to get going and even the smallest of tasks seem insurmountable.

The outcome of not being able to solve these simple problems starts to grow into large problems, which leads into more anxiety and depression. When you are emotionally distressed you find that nearly everything seems to be overwhelmingly hard and this is because emotional pain will interfere with your clear thinking.

When you are feeling overwhelmed you begin to avoid any situation or problem and start to procrastinate for as long as you can. **Avoidance of the problem is not going to make the problem go away, it will only make it worse.**

Below are nine ways you can deal with these problems head on:

1. **Avoid wallowing in your problems.** Is there a specific situation that

is causing you to feel down? If there is, you need to avoid dwelling on this problem/situation. Identify the problem and it's causes; what are your beliefs and feelings about this problem? The next step is to work out possible solutions so that you can address the problem. If this seems too hard to do at times then shift your mind to something that makes you happy and come back to solving this another time.

2. **Keep busy with things you enjoy.** In your free time, why not do the things you like? By selecting activities you enjoy will make this process a lot easier than trying something you do not enjoy. Find something that will put that smile back on your face.

3. **Seek out the company of others.** At times you may get down because you feel lonely. There is always someone out there that you can spend some time with, even if it's not one of your

close friends. Work out which activity you would both enjoy doing or simply just sit and have a good chat.

4. **Pursue a new hobby.** Are you bored? Consider starting up a new hobby that you have always wanted to do, who knows where this new activity might lead you.

5. **Take a class.** Learning something new is always a great way to take your mind off your problems. Why not pick a subject that you have interest in and sign up. You will find that your new class will stir up some great excitement that will put your problems in the background.

6. **Meet new people.** Meeting new people is always good for you, in more ways than you can imagine. You can find new people to chat with everywhere. You can even do it without leaving your home by finding like-minded people online. Meeting a new

friend that you connect well with can certainly improve your mood.

7. **Start new adventures.** Starting a new adventure is a wonderful way of connecting with your friends and family. If you prefer to be alone, you can always go on a solo adventure. Let your mind go wild with fun ideas. Your feelings of sadness will disappear as you begin planning an exciting new adventure.

8. **Activate your muscles.** By being more active in your daily routine certainly has benefits to help you feel better about you and your life. A walk in the fresh air for instance can be uplifting for your mood.

   Your emotional mindset might tell you that you don't feel like it or you're too tired, but chances are that once you get moving, you'll be glad that you went out of your way to get some exercise.

9. **Get in touch with your spiritual side.** This is always something that some people just do not even think about, but seriously it can be beneficial to you. Even if you are not a religious person you can contemplate the answers to life's big questions. When you focus on the big picture, sometimes your own challenges don't feel as large anymore.

The next time you feel down make a real effort to try just one of these tips – it may be just the thing to help you turn that frown upside down!

Chapter Affirmation:

I find happiness everywhere I look.

When I look around me, I see happiness. **Even when there are trying times, there is always happiness to be found.** *Every cloud really does have a silver lining, and I take the time to find it.*

Happiness is a state of mind. If I expect to see happiness, I do. Unlike too many others who expect to see sadness, I expect happiness and joy. Because I look for good things, I see good things. Sadness has no place in my life.

My mind is focused on things that make me happy. *Joy can be simple or complex, but it is always available to everyone, including me.*

Even though things might be imperfect, there is value in every situation. ***There is always something to be happy about.*** *Even breathing is a gift, because it shows I am still alive. There is happiness in that gift for anyone who is willing to see it.*

I am always willing to see happiness instead of sadness. ***The ability to find happiness is within me.***

When I look, I see happiness in my life
and in the lives of others. Because I see
happiness, I am able to share what I see
with others. This helps me bring joy to the
lives of other people.

Today, I look carefully around me to see
the happiness in everything.

Self-Reflection Questions:

1. How can I see more happiness in my
   life?
2. Can I find ways to help others see
   more happiness in their own lives?
3. What can I do to share my own joy
   with others?

Chapter Fifteen

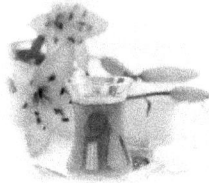

Heal Your Body With Relaxation Techniques

"Relaxation means releasing all concern and tension and letting the natural order of life flow through one's being" –
Donald Curtis

When you struggle with anxiety and depression it is always good to know that there are natural ways to help you relieve your suffering.

It is very important that you breathe deeply and fully as this helps your body stay calm. You may still feel tense, however this deep breathing can help protect you against an anxiety attack. With an anxiety attack you tend to hyperventilate and this increases the level of panic that you will experience, the deep breathing will help you keep this in control.

Concentrate on your breathing by making sure you breathe all the way down to your abdomen, this will help improve your relaxation to any stressful situations.

Following are breathing techniques that are beneficial:

Place a hand just above your belly button and breathe. If you're breathing deeply, your hand will rise and fall with each breath.

Practice breathing slowly by taking full, deep breaths. You might feel a bit strange at first because you're not used to it. You may even feel a bit giddy, but that's normal. This will pass with practice.

You're getting plenty of air, even if you don't feel like you are. It is important to note that your lungs can expand without your upper chest rising. Only your upper belly needs to rise and fall. At first, you probably won't breathe this way unless you're thinking about it because you're so conditioned to breathe from your chest. ***Keep practicing often, and you'll soon be breathing properly all the time.***

Understanding How Breathing Affects Anxiety

It is understood that anxiety may be caused by a chemical imbalance in the brain that may simply be the product of over-active nerves that react too strongly to stimuli. No matter what causes you to feel anxious, the most important thing is to be able to alleviate it and to reduce the degree to which it affects your life.

By lowering your anxiety, you may be able to:

- Change careers or get promoted
- Speak in front of others without fear
- Travel to places you've always wanted to see
- Embark on a new relationship or business venture
- Reduce your dependency on medication or therapy

Remember that you need to consult your doctor before changing any type of medication or therapy, however these breathing exercises can be implemented right away as they are natural and will not result in any side effects.

Another Beneficial Technique That You Can Implement is Meditation

Meditation is a beneficial self-help technique that can help you to get in touch with yourself. Meditation can help you to relieve stress, relax you body, as well as calming your mind.

Pick a time of the day when you will not get any interruptions and set this time aside for your meditation. Begin your meditation by taking deep breathes and focusing only on each breath as it goes in and out.

Some days you may be stressed and have difficulty focusing on your breathing. When this happens acknowledge the thought that comes and then go back to concentrating on your breathing. You will feel calm if you keep this up.

As your mind becomes calm, start to take notice of the thoughts that do come into play, but only notice them, nothing else; quickly return your attention back to your breathing. If any of these thoughts make you tense or uncomfortable, just relax your muscles and return to your breathing again.

By practising this meditation, it will get easier and you will enjoy and look forward to your relaxation time.

Chapter Affirmation:

I am the body in motion that stays in motion.

This universal law of physics applies to both my body and mind. Once I start an activity, it's easy to maintain momentum. Knowing this, I can soar past obstacles in my path and remain focused on my tasks and goals.

I create my action plans so they begin with undemanding tasks. This allows me to start any project with ease. Then I can quickly complete that task and move effortlessly onto the next, gaining momentum as I move forward.

The energy of my forward momentum helps push challenges aside. *My active and focused mind is able to figure out a way to work with or overcome difficulties. Sometimes I may have to alter my plans, but I always maintain momentum.*

It is similar to a game of pool. Once the cue hits the ball with enough energy to give it a strong push, it continues its momentum regardless of anything in its path. When it hits another ball or the wall, it simply changes its path and keeps going.

Like the ball, each and every day I have a chance to take my turn and do with it what I will! I choose to maintain my forward momentum with my eyes on my prize, even if I must change my plan from time to time.

Just as the ball comes to a stop at the end of its turn, **I wind down at the end of the day and rest.** *The next morning I*

125

feel rejuvenated and I have the energy to take another exciting turn in this wonderful game of life!

Today, I strive to be the body in motion that stays in motion. With my forward momentum, I can handle anything that steers me away from my tasks. I may change my route to overcome challenges that arise, but I am still on course to attain my goals.

Self-Reflection Questions:

1. Do I include easy tasks at the start of my action plans?
2. What challenges in my life do I allow to stop my momentum?
3. Can I alter my path to get past my challenges so I can keep moving forward?

Chapter Sixteen

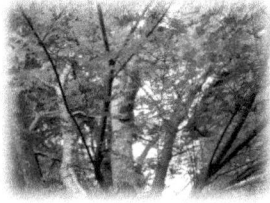

Notes On

Medication

"There is no such thing in anyone's life as an unimportant day" - Alexander Woollcott

Please understand that the information in this chapter is not a substitute for medical advice; please consult with your medical professional about your own personal requirements.

Anxiety and Depression disorders can be treated effectively, it is vital that you consult and discuss your circumstances with your medical professional. If you are someone that is experiencing feelings of sadness that has been going on for some time or it is effecting your life in a great way then you need to seek medical help.

The treatment that you require will depend on your symptoms, however the following are some of the treatments available to you:

1. There are psychological interventions like cognitive behavioural therapy (CBT) that is specially aimed at changing patterns of thinking, behaviour and beliefs that are related to depression.
2. Anti-depressant medications that help to relieve depressed feelings, restore appetite and normal sleep patterns, as well as reduce anxiety. Anti-depressants are not addictive like tranquillisers; they help to slowly return the balance of neuro-transmitters in your brain. You can

usually see positive results from between one to four weeks.

3. Therapy and self-help strategies are very beneficial to help you get to the real issues so that you can develop the tools that will help you overcome anxiety for good.

4. There are specific medications that can help you with your mood swings, for example bipolar disorder. Please see your medical professional to see which one is best suited to your specific needs.

5. In some cases a lifestyle change can be very beneficial. Adding an exercise regime will greatly increase your changes of recovery. The reduction of alcohol and harmful drugs can help with your recovery from depression as well.

6. If you have a severe form of depression then your medical professional may suggest electroconvulsive therapy (ECT). This can be a life saving treatment for people that are at a high risk of suicide

or in the case of the severity of this illness causing you to stop eating or drinking which can cause death.

There are many different types of medications available for the treatment of anxiety disorders like the traditional anti-anxiety drug called benzodiazepine or the more recent medications called antidepressants and beta-blockers.

Even though these medications can be effective they are not the ultimate cure, it will give you temporary relief but it will not fix the underlying problem of your anxiety disorder. Once medications are halted your anxiety symptoms will return in full swing.

It is vital that you seek professional advice not only on what medication you specifically need but also what treatment is required for the underlying issues to your disorder. Remember that in most instances you need to treat your anxiety disorder with medication and a therapy option that is best suited to your specific situation.

Chapter Affirmation:

I enjoy each day despite my health challenges.

*Even with a health challenge, I have much joy each day. Challenges are there to be met and handled. I experience joy when I overcome obstacles and achieve success in any way. **As long as I have life, I have joy.***

I do what I am capable of doing and I allow that to be enough. Small joys take on more significance during the holidays. I let those joys carry me through any challenge.

*Reflecting on each day keeps me sustained throughout the year. I look forward to the next day. **Each day brings something new and wonder-***

ful into my life. I choose to let go of anger and blame over my health. I accept my reality so I can move forward with joy and peace.

Staying in peace through every day is important to me. **I have many joyous events in my life.** *I choose happiness in spite of anything that others might find troubling. My happiness and joy are my greatest holiday gifts to other people. I give them my joy willingly.*

If times are difficult, I release any fear or anxiety. **I am alive and that is what matters.** *I have people who love and care for me, and we celebrate our time together. We all make memories that last a lifetime. These memories bring me a lot of contentment and comfort as I face my health challenges during each and every day.*

Today, I choose happiness and joy for every day of my life regardless of my challenges.

Self-Reflection Questions:

1. *How can I get more joy from each day?*
2. *What can I do to feel better about the health challenges I face?*
3. *Are there ways I can reach out to encourage others with health challenges?*

Chapter Seventeen

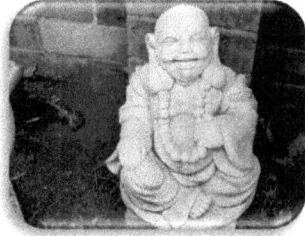

Improving Your

Relationships &

Avoiding Conflicts

"What you are is what you have been, and what you will be is what you do now" - Buddha

Having supportive relationships are essential in life at all times not just when you are having emotional distress issues. Research has shown that by having good supportive relationships whether it is from friends, family or strangers can help improve your mental and physical health immensely.

Humans are programmed biologically to function better when they are surrounded by supportive relationships. By improving your relationships you can help yourself to boost your mood, enhance your general well-being and the ability to increase your handle on stress.

When you are depressed your emotions can hinder all of your relationships and can cause irreversible damage, so it is very important that you concentrate on improving your relationships so that you can use this tool when you are feeling down, the support of these relationships can help you to lift your mood and allow you to defeat anxiety and depression.

It is only natural that you become self-absorbed when you are depressed or anxious, some people may think that you are being selfish, however that is not the case, you are just focused on your problems and concerns. It is understood that the focus of your attention is on your problems and that your relationships will suffer in the process as your energy is shifted from them to your problems and concerns.

What happens when you are in this state is that you become emotionally and mentally drained so you do not pay attention to your relationships, however this is where you need to remember that you need to keep working on improving your relationships.

Another important point to remember is that when you are anxious and depressed, your friends and family will try to help you and when they don't get any response after persisting they will soon turn away from you because they feel frustrated and helpless. Eventually these people will withdraw from you completely and this is understandable but is not the ideal end result that you need.

Following are some ways on how you can improve your relationship with someone that has anxiety and depression:

- Remember to take care of yourself
- Get the support required
- Educate yourself about anxiety and depression
- Always be there for them
- Remember not to take their actions personally
- Offer plenty of hope
- Get the treatment that they need
- Like dogs, learn to love them unconditionally
- Help them by taking the pressure off

It is very important that you avoid conflicts with anyone if you are anxious or depressed. It will not help you and can cause you to become more irritable which only results in a greater conflict.

When you are anxious, depressed or are in conflict with someone you feel more emotionally vulnerable, so it becomes too easy to jump to negative conclusions. When you are in this state of mind you automatically have negative assumptions and you miss the true meaning of what is being said.

Following are the results of a conflict:

- Conflicts can trigger strong emotions
- Conflicts will continue to fester if they are ignored
- Conflicts are more than just a disagreement with someone
- Conflicts are responded to based on our perception of the situation
- Conflicts can be used as an opportunity for growth

The best way you can avoid conflict is to implement the following:

- Remain in control of your emotions and behaviour
- Understand and respect that there are differences

- Master the management of your stress so that you can remain calm and alert at all times
- Understand the feelings being expressed by the other person and don't take it personally

It is really important that you improve your relationships and avoid all conflicts whenever possible, this will not only help you but it will allow you to build on the relationships that are important to you and your health.

<u>Chapter Affirmation:</u>

My family triumphs through trouble.

Every family, including mine, experiences hardships. It's only natural to have personalities clash in a home with so many strong-minded individuals.

When my children have a negative attitude towards my partner and I, we take it with a grain of salt. Their temperamen-

tal behavior is temporary and simply a sign of growth. **I remember how we were once just as stubborn as our children** and felt as if our parents were enemies. I understand that they're just going through a phase.

Though it may seem at times like our family fights a lot, **our bond is undeniably strong.**

In the past, my spouse and I took spending time with our children for granted; now we savor every moment spent by their side. Nothing feels better than my daughter asking, "Hey mum, want to go to the mall?" She could have asked any of her friends to go with her, but she asked me!

My spouse and I raise them to the best of our abilities, and we wholeheartedly believe that we are doing a stupendous job! Sure, my partner and I have our differences. But, who doesn't? **We are two separate individuals, with wholly**

separate opinions. *I value my partner for voicing his thoughts, beliefs, and ideas.*

Regardless of our differences, my partner and I remain strong throughout the years. We triumph through troubles, as does our entire family. Each battle makes us stronger. Each scar is a memory of the long way we've come. And, **each tear is a sign of a lesson learned.**

Today, I accept my family for the strong individuals we are. Raising children and simultaneously maintaining a marriage has its challenges. But, we've managed to triumph through all of our troubles.

Self-Reflection Questions:

1. *How can we carve out more family time?*
2. *Am I supportive of my family's growth?*
3. *Which defining moments have we experienced as a family?*

Chapter Eighteen

How To Avoid A

Repeat

Performance

"It is hard to fail, but it is worse never to have tried to succeed" –
Theodore Roosevelt

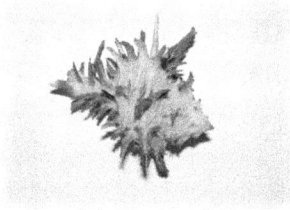

Avoiding a repeat performance is possible because anxiety and depression can both be treated effectively. It is important that you keep working on the treatment or therapy that is helping you to improve. If

143

you find that these treatments or therapies are no longer working effectively, then you need to change to something else, please make sure that you do this with the advice of your medical professional.

By maintaining your treatment/therapies you will put yourself in a better position to avoid a repeat performance.

Following is a worksheet to help you avoid a repeat performance:

Print out this checklist and try these methods of stopping or preventing your panic attacks. Track your results by marking off each tip when you use it and take note whether or not it made a difference in your life.

Remember, with a determined mindset, you can overcome a panic attack!

Tip	Have I used this tip?	Was this tip help-ful?
Meditate first thing each morning.	**YES NO**	**YES NO**
Squeeze an anti-stress ball or slide oriental therapeutic balls between your palms.	**YES NO**	**YES NO**
Practice deep breathing exercises until you feel your nerves relaxing.	**YES NO**	**YES NO**

Focus your energy on an activity that requires all of your attention, like sending an email, solving a Sudoku puzzle or mowing the lawn.	**YES NO**	**YES NO**
Play a recording of positive statements.	**YES NO**	**YES NO**

Slowly recite your ABCs, while saying a word that starts with the corresponding letter.	**YES NO**	**YES NO**
Listen to a song that allows you to reflect on happy memories, such as your wedding day or your child's birth.	**YES NO**	**YES NO**

Laugh at yourself. Turning the situation into a comedy-fest rather than a fear-fest will bring about positive emotions.	**YES NO**	**YES NO**
Call your spouse in the beginning stages of your panic attack. Hearing their voice just might help you relax.	**YES NO**	**YES NO**

Write down what happens after each panic attack. Remind yourself that you're not in danger when experiencing a panic attack.	**YES NO**	**YES NO**
Avoid caffeine and sugary/energy drinks. These drinks make you highly excitable.	**YES NO**	**YES NO**

Face your fears. Once you do, you'll realise that you have nothing to worry about and no person, place, or thing is a "bad luck charm."	**YES NO**	**YES NO**
Sleep 6 to 8 hours each night. Lack of sleep makes you more prone to panic attacks.	**YES NO**	**YES NO**

Repeat, *"If I relax, I'll be able to continue my day normally within a few seconds."*	**YES NO**	**YES NO**
For each minute that you allow yourself to endure a panic attack, force yourself to run, iron clothes, or do another task for 10 minutes.	**YES NO**	**YES NO**

Time your panic attacks. Each time you shave 2 minutes off of your last recorded duration, reward yourself with a nice dinner or treat.	YES NO	YES NO

Chapter Affirmation:

Sharing love with others makes me joyful.

My heart, mind, and spirit are full of love. I enjoy sharing that love with the people around me. By my words and actions, people see that I have a lot of love to give. **Love is important to the world, and I do my part to pass it on to others.**

I take great joy from sharing my love with other people. Even a smile can make someone happy, so I take the time to smile at people and give them a kind word. I am happiest when I am sharing my love instead of keeping it all for myself.

Love is a gift to be shared. *Sharing love is the best way to get love to come into my life. When I give love, I get love* back. I reap the benefits, and so do others.

There is so much joy in treating others with love and kindness. It affects the way I feel and brings positive energy to me. Because I receive positive energy, I have more love to pass on to more people. **Love grows and grows because I water it daily.**

I continue to encourage others to spread love and joy. Encouragement is important, and many people need what I have to offer. By helping others to love, I help myself, as well. As I freely offer love to more people, it spreads like ripples in a pond, eventually reaching everyone.

Today, I share my love of life with everyone around me.

Self-Reflection Questions:

1. *How can I bring more love into my own life?*
2. *What can I do to share my love of life with others?*
3. *How can I encourage others to have a more loving attitude?*

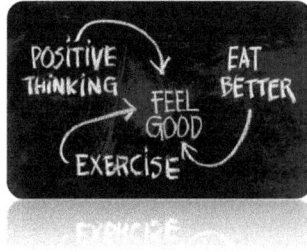

Chapter Nineteen

How To Remain Positive

"People often say that motivation doesn't last. Well, neither does bathing. That's why we recommend it daily" - Zig Ziglar

It is vital to your health and well being to remain positive. By implementing the tips and tools in this book you can overcome your anxiety and depression. It is possible, I have done it and so can you. You deserve to feel better just like me. You can achieve true happiness once more!

There has been many studies and research done on how happiness not only makes you feel good, but being happy helps your immune system, lowers your blood pressure, longevity and allows you to feel empathy for our fellow human being.

People that are happy are more successful, productive and satisfied with life in general. If that is not enough for you to strive for happiness then I don't know what is!

Gratitude is a wonderful thing and is the one thing that really helps you with your happiness and your well-being. By concentrating on all the good in your life and being really aware of what gives you that wonderful feeling of gratitude is amazingly helpful in developing your overall sense of well-being.

A few powerful things that you can implement to help you achieve wonderful happiness are:

- Being good to others
- Letting go of grudges and anger
- Having complete self control
- Figuring out what is important in your life
- Being grateful for all that surrounds you

Make a list of what you are grateful for and read them out aloud each day. Please find the following affirmations as a guideline to help you create your own list:

1.   I feel an abundance of gratitude for everything I have and receive every day.

2.   My needs and desires are generously met. For this I am thankful.

3.   I am grateful for all the great health, love, and goodness that my life has revealed to me.

4.   I am continually amazed at how abundant my life is already!

5.   I am grateful for everything I experience

in this lifetime. I overcome, I grow, and I prosper all the time. My abundant blessings, as well as my difficulties, all make me better, stronger, and more alive.

6.   I am so grateful for every person and every thing in my life.

7.   I appreciate everything I have and I show my sincerest gratitude to my loved ones.

8.   The universe pours joy into my life every day. It has my cup overflowing with wealth, health, and love.

9.   My life is singular, unique and wondrous. For this I am profoundly thankful.

10.   I clearly see the beauty of life that flourishes around me.

11.   I give gratitude for God's endless treasures.

12.   I am grateful for my blessed ancestors living on through my blood.

Using the affirmations above along with your own will help you lead a less stressful and more fulfilling life.

Spending some time with positive affirmations, while appreciating all that you have and all that's heading your way is one of the easiest "stress relief drugs" you'll ever take. Yet, affirmations come with no ill side effects and they're free. Choose peace in your life by using the power of affirmations and gratitude, it truly will help you, I am happy to say they helped me personally in a huge way that I thought was never even possible!

Chapter Affirmation:

I have many reasons to live.

I love life! When I wake up in the morning, I am thankful to be alive and healthy. Every day, I have dozens of reasons to get out of my bed and live my life to the fullest.

My family needs me to be my best for them. Even when they have trouble communicating their love to me or when we fail to agree, my family loves me and needs me. **I matter to my family.**

My friends enjoy my company. I have a personality and a sense of humor that is irreplaceable. My friends love being around me and look forward to spending time with me. **I am loved and accepted by my friends.**

The work I perform at my job is important to many people. **I am the only one in the world who can do my job quite like me.** *My co-workers and superiors miss me when I am absent from work. I am indispensable!*

I look forward to living a long, happy, and healthy life. My future is bright! I am at peace with what life holds for me and I anticipate what is to come with joy.

I visualise myself traveling the world, experiencing many amazing things, and accomplishing unbelievable dreams. ***I see myself demolishing the barriers that surround me today.***

Today, I count my blessings and give thanks for my life. Living one day at a time, I remind myself that the storms of life pass by, giving way to serene peace.

Self-Reflection Questions:

1. *How can I reconnect with my loved ones?*
2. *When was the last time I was victorious over a difficult situation?*
3. *What am I most looking forward to in the future?*

Chapter Twenty

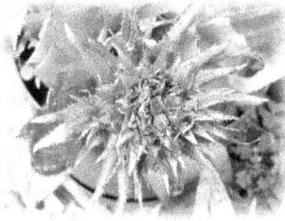

How To Keep Your Mood Alive & Well!

"Your time is limited, so don't waste it living someone else's life" - Steve Jobs

I understand that overcoming your anxiety and depression does not happen overnight, it takes time and most of all persistence when you don't feel like it, but you need to always have it in the back of your mind that you can do this, no matter how hard times get, you will come through at the other end and be that happy soul that you once were. I did it and so can you!

I have compiled some uplifting affirmations that helped me and I want to share them with you so that you too can have the same if not better results than I did.

50 affirmations to keep your mood alive and well:

1. I am willing to begin with an open heart and mind
2. I give myself permission to be calm
3. I am strong and competent
4. I can tame my fears because I am in control
5. When I feel anxious, I ask fact finding questions and I know I am on solid ground
6. I let go of the feeling of being in unknown territory
7. I have no need to worry about the unknown. I enjoy living in the moment

8. My mistakes make me stronger. I learn from them.
9. I no longer need to be frightened. I allow myself to receive the light of who I am
10. I can accept uncertainty when it comes
11. Worry and anxiety cannot change my circumstance, only positive thoughts and actions can
12. I can remove the blindfold of anxiety and focus on the gold at the end of the rainbow
13. I am fully capable of managing any challenge that comes my way
14. I am not afraid. I love my new feelings of calm and joy
15. When I keep moving in the right direction, I feel calm
16. I can remain calm in times of change
17. I do not sweat on the small stuff
18. I challenge myself to be calm in order to release daily pressures
19. I am not perfect and that's okay

20. Uncertainty does not sway me from my plan of action
21. The more I let go of unrealistic comparisons, the better I feel
22. I am excited by the presence of a new day
23. I am a problem solver
24. I grow more patient with myself and others everyday
25. I let go of others' opinions of me. It doesn't matter what they think
26. I accept people as they are
27. I avoid focusing on the trees so I don't lose sight of the lush, beautiful forest before me
28. I am relinquishing control over the uncontrollable
29. I am comfortable with the set of challenges a new day brings
30. It is easy for me to let go and enjoy the laughter I have inside of me
31. My life is full of peace and happiness
32. I find reasons to laugh everyday
33. I am where I want to be in life

34. I am thankful for all opportunities. My attitude reflects my happiness
35. I open myself to experience all feelings
36. I am happy with myself. I relax and enjoy my life
37. I enjoy being me!
38. I savour each moment of each day
39. In order to share happiness with others, I must also be happy
40. There is a beautiful light at the end of the tunnel
41. I give myself permission to be happy
42. I choose not to allow unnecessary stress to control me. I deserve peace.
43. I trust my ability to relax. I am calm and peaceful.
44. I know that healing my mind gives me more energy to tackle new challenges
45. I relax to get my mind off the things that I cannot control
46. Situations do not control me

47. It is safe for me to release the imaginary constraints that I have placed on my life
48. No matter how I'm feeling, I simply begin. I am able to build momentum to accomplish anything
49. I am at peace with others because I choose to interact well each time
50. I allow all of my tension to leave my body right away

Replenish your mind, body and soul each and every day by reading these out aloud.

I know that these affirmations are probably enough in one chapter, however I really thought that this one below was one that you would enjoy regardless!

Chapter Affirmation:

I am captivated by my life.

Because I recognise that life is fleeting, I focus on making each minute count. I work hard to create the most fascinating, fun, and educational life I can make for myself. I look for ways to be enthralled with my daily activities. I am captivated by my life.

Living an entrancing life means I am never bored. *Even when I rest, I engage in activities that bring me joy. Simple pleasures such as reading the news or watching an old episode of a beloved comedy show brings quiet satisfaction.*

Listening to music captures and holds my attention. I am interested in the stories behind the songs. Everything I do enriches my life. Each of my activities delights me.

171

When I get to spend time with my family members or friends, I am entranced by the whole experience.

Being surrounded by people I love, who also love me, is fulfilling and brings feelings of deep satisfaction. In these situations, I am once again captivated by my own life.

A continuing goal for me is to experience contentment, delight and sheer pleasure each day. I embrace everything positive that comes my way as I release everything else. Doing this helps me to love my life.

Today, I reflect on my life and appreciate how it continually brings me joy and delight, captivating me with its thrills.

Self-Reflection Questions:

4. *Am I enamored of my life?*
5. *What parts of my life bring joy, fascination and delight? What aspects of my life bring me down?*
6. *How can I ensure I consistently live a captivating life?*

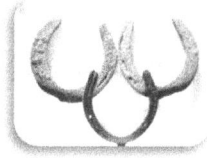

Chapter Twenty One

Anxiety & Depression Checklist & Worksheet

"Don't cheat the world of your contribution. Give it what you've got" – Steven Pressfield

1. Do I talk about my feelings? To whom?

2. Am I in a constant state of worry?
   What am I worried about?

3. Am I giving power to my anxious
   thoughts?
   What will I do to put my worries
   into perspective?

4. Is my routine contributing to my
   depression or anxiety?
   What will I change to improve my
   health?

5. Am I plagued by negative
   thoughts?
   What will I do to introduce positive thoughts into my life?

6. Do I bottle up my thoughts and
   feelings?
   What will I do to release this pressure?

7. Do I feel alone? Who can I seek for help?

Chapter Affirmation:

My life has remarkable worth.

I am an individual created for a grand purpose. I am the only one in this world who can do what I am called to do.

There are people who love me more than they are able to express. *My family, my friends, and my colleagues think the world of me. Even if we fail to see eye to eye at times, they still have great respect for me.*

Even when I feel overlooked by others, I am still valuable. Many people notice my work, and those people may never get the chance to tell me. Life moves fast and some people simply don't take the time to tell me that they notice my work.

My worth lies in my own view of myself. When I acknowledge that my Creator designed me for a noble purpose, my confidence grows.

My destiny is just waiting for me to fulfill it. There are amazing things in my future, which I work hard to attain. **I refuse to allow discouragement to rob me of my destiny.**

I am precious to my Creator. Even when it is hard for me to see my own worth, I know that I am valuable. Each morning, I turn the page of my past and embrace the new chance to make a change.

Today, I choose to see myself as a chest filled with treasure. I have more beauty than diamonds and more worth than gold.

Self-Reflection Questions:

1. *Do I ever feel invisible?*
2. *Do I acknowledge my worth?*
3. *Why does my life matter? To whom does my life matter?*

About The Author

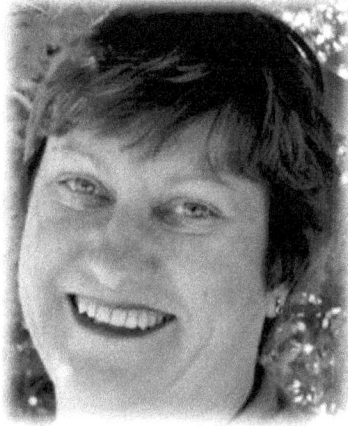

Sue Kennedy is an author and consultant. Her first book Defeat Diabetes Now is all about how you can reverse diabetes naturally. Sue wrote this book to help her mother that was diagnosed with diabetes, because of the success her mum had, she now has a website where she sells her book to help others.

Apart from her own experiences with Anxiety and Depression, she has written this book to help people that are first diagnosed with diabetes plus people that develop this terrible illness of anxiety and depression that can be caused by so many other troubles and situations.

Her ultimate goal is to help people get back on track with their health and well-being so that they can live the life that they deserve. If you would like more information please visit her website at http://www.DefeatDiabetesNow.com.au.

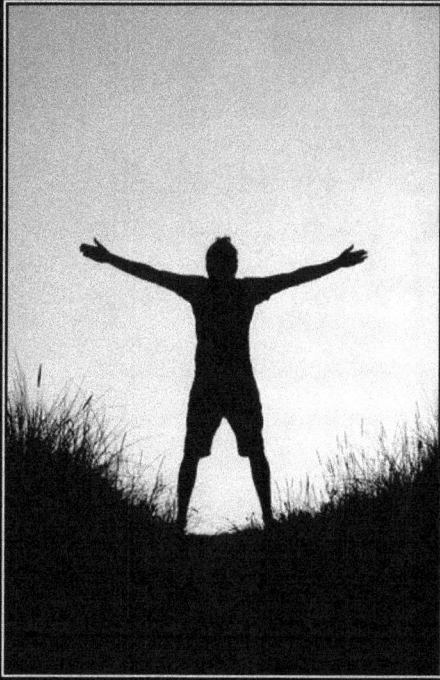

I AM HAPPY

My Life Is Full Of Abundance

www.ingramcontent.com/pod-product-compliance
Lightning Source LLC
Chambersburg PA
CBHW060852280326
41934CB00007B/1011